CUMIN

MARIAN KIM

ISBN: 1508574928

ISBN-13: 978-1508574927

CONTENTS

MARIAN KIM

1

PROPERTIES

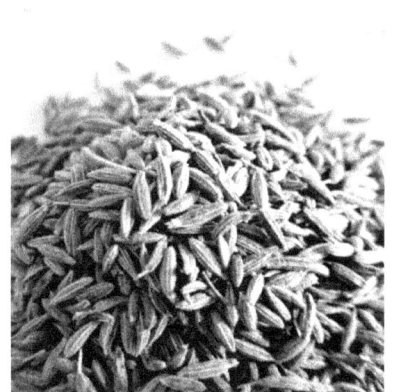

Scientific name: Cuminum cyminum

Other names: Anis acre, jeeraka

Nutrients: Iron and manganese

Properties

Anti-oxidant properties which protect the cells from free radical damage that causes degenerative diseases and premature aging

Anti-aging properties

Anti-cancer properties

Carminative (anti-flatulent) properties

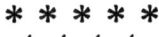

2

USES

Heart attack and stroke prevention

A study found that cumin prevents platelets from sticking together and forming clots and thus may therefore prevent strokes and heart attacks.

Weight loss

Cumin is used for weight loss since it aids the production of energy by the body.

Memory enhancement

Cumin is used for brain health since a study found that it protects against memory loss. It also confers protection from the harmful effects of stress on the body.

Stress management

Cumin helps a person manage stress better.

Fluid retention

Cumin acts as a diuretic and is used for fluid retention.

Flatulence treatment

Cumin tea is used to treat flatulence (intestinal gas).

Upset stomach treatment

Cumin is also used to treat upset stomachs.

Anorexia treatment

Cumin seeds chewed before a meal can stimulate the appetite.

Digestive aid

Cumin is used as a digestive aid since it stimulates the productions of pancreatic enzymes.

Crampy abdominal pain treatment

Ground cumin mixed with honey is used to relieve intestinal cramps and colic pain.

Parasite abdominal pain treatment

Cumin poultice is used to relieve abdominal pain caused by intestinal parasites.

Loose stools treatment

Ground cumin mixed with honey is used to reduce loose stools due to poor digestion.

Irritable Bowel Syndrome (IBS) relief

Roasted cumin seeds are mixed with pomegranate juice and used to relieve IBS symptoms like frequent stools. These seeds should be roasted very briefly to prevent the evaporation of the healing oils.

Hemorrhoid relief

One teaspoon of gently roasted cumin seeds can be pureed with a ¼ inch slice of ginger and a pinch of salt and drunk with butter milk to soothe inflamed hemorrhoids.

Amenorrhea

Cumin stimulates menstruation.

Morning sickness relief

Ground cumin added to lime juice is used to relieve morning sickness.

Induce milk production

Cumin infusions can be taken to stimulate milk production in nursing mothers.

Breast swellings

Cumin poultices are used to treat breast swellings.

Testicle swellings

Cumin poultices are used to treat testicle swellings.

Cutaneous boils relief

Cumin seeds mixed with water to make a paste are used to reduce the pain and inflammation of boils.

Insect sting relief

Cumin seeds mixed with water to make a paste are used to reduce the pain and inflammation of insect stings.

Nose bleed treatment

Cumin nasal drops made by mixing cumin tea with vinegar are used to treat nose bleeding.

Oral ulcers relief

Cumin tea mixed with some cardamom is used as a gargle to aid in the healing of sores in the mouth.

Gingivitis relief

Cumin tea mixed with some cardamom is used as a gargle to aid in the healing of bleeding gums. Gently roasted cumin seeds can also be ground and mixed with salt to create a powder to massage the gums and prevent gingivitis.

Hiccup treatment

Cumin with ghee is smoked to treat hiccups.

Common cold relief

Cumin tea with a slice of ginger can be used to relieve the symptoms of the common cold.

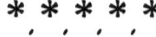

3

SAFETY PRECAUTIONS

1. Persons scheduled to have surgery should stop taking cumin 2 weeks before the operation since it might lower blood sugar levels during and after the surgery.

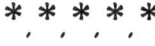

4

DRUG INTERACTIONS

1. Cumin can interact with diabetes medications and lower blood sugar levels.

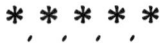

5

COOKING TIPS

Flavor: Rich smoky

Food pairing: Vegetables e.g. cucumbers and tomatoes, fruits e.g. avocados, mangos and citrus fruits, meat dishes e.g. beef, coconuts, grains, poultry, fish, seafood, sausages, beans

Blends well with: Cilantro, garlic, mint, onion, parsley

Can be substituted with: Chili powder

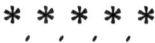

6

HERBAL RECIPES

Cumin Tea

Equipment

Kettle

Tea cup

***

Ingredients

1 teaspoon of finely crushed cumin

1 cup of boiling water

Honey to taste (optional)

***

Instructions

1. Put the cumin in a tea cup, add the boiling water and let it steep while covered for 10 -15 minutes.

2. Add honey (if using) to suit your taste before drinking.

*****

Cumin Infusion

Equipment

Glass jar with tight fitting lid

***

Ingredients

1 tablespoon cumin

1 cup boiling water

***

Instructions

1. Place the cumin in the glass jar and add the boiling water to fill the jar.

2. Close the lid and let the mixture steep for 4 hours to 14 hours (overnight).

3. Strain the cumin and the infusion is ready for consumption.

***

Tips

1. Store the infusion in the refrigerator to lengthen its life.

*****

Cumin Syrup

Equipment

Saucepan

Jar with airtight lid

***

Ingredients

1 quart (1000 ml) filtered water

1 cup cumin

1 cup honey

***

Instructions

1. Place the water and cumin in a saucepan and bring to a boil.

2. Reduce the heat and let it simmer while it is partially covered until the volume is reduced to half the original volume.

3. Strain the mixture through a sieve or cheesecloth to remove the cumin.

4. Measure 1 pint (500 mls) of the liquid and add the honey.

5. Cook for a few minutes as you stir it so that it thickens.

6. Store the syrup in an airtight container in the fridge for up to 2 months.

*****

Cumin Poultice

Equipment

Cheesecloth or old cotton sheet strips

***

Ingredients

1 tablespoon cumin powder

Boiling water

***

Instructions

1. Add enough boiling water to the cumin powder to wet it and make a thick paste.

2. Spoon the cumin paste onto the cheesecloth (or bed sheet strips) to make the poultice.

3. To use, apply the poultice to the affected area and cover with another piece of hot, wet cloth. Replace the hot, wet cloth when it cools with another hot one to keep the poultice hot.

*****

Cumin Tincture

Equipment

Glass jar with tight fitting lid

Dark tincture bottles

Cheesecloth

Labels

***

Ingredients

7 oz (200 gm) cumin

30 oz (1 liter) of 80-100 proof vodka

***

Instructions

1. Fill 1/3 of the glass jar with the cumin.

2. Add the vodka to completely fill the jar to the top.

3. Seal the jar and label it with the date of preparation and name of spice used. Store the glass jar in a dark place for 6 weeks ensuring that you shake them weekly.

4. After 6 weeks strain out the cumin with a cheesecloth and pour the tincture into dark tincture bottles.

5. Label the tincture bottles and store your cumin tinctures away from light and heat.

*****

Cumin Infused Oil

Equipment

Double boiler

Large glass bowl

Sieve and cheesecloth

Sterilized dark jars

***

Ingredients

16 fl oz. (500 ml) vegetable oil like olive or sweet almond oil

8 oz. (250 grams) slightly crushed cumin

***

Instructions

1. Place the cumin and oil in the glass bowl ensuring that the oil covers the spice. Simmer them in a double boiler for 1 hour at 120 degrees Fahrenheit (49 degrees Celsius). Do not let the mixture boil. You can repeat this step after letting the oils cool to create more concentrated spice infused oils.

2. Strain the mixture through the sieve and cheesecloth into a clean, dark jar ensuring you squeeze out as much oil as you can from the cheesecloth.

3. Label your jars with the manufacturing date, expiry date, spice and oils used. Store your cumin infused oils in a cool dark place or in the refrigerator and use them within 3 months.

*****

Cumin Butter

Equipment

Large glass bowl

Electric mixer or stick blender or wire whisk

Molds such as ice cube trays (optional)

***

Ingredients

½ cup butter

2 tablespoons of finely crushed cumin

***

Instructions

1. Place the butter in a warm place so that it can soften.

2. Put butter and cumin in a large glass bowl and blend well until thoroughly mixed.

3. Refrigerate until it hardens. You can refrigerate it in molds or ice cube trays to give it a special shape.

###

ABOUT THE AUTHOR

Marian Kim is an experienced alternative medicine practitioner.

*****

OTHER BOOKS BY THE AUTHOR

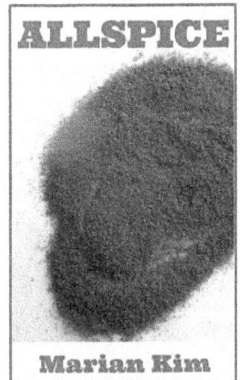

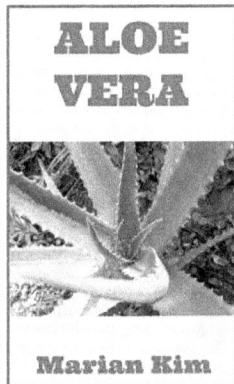

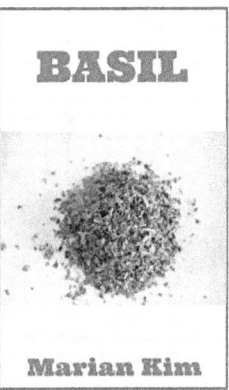

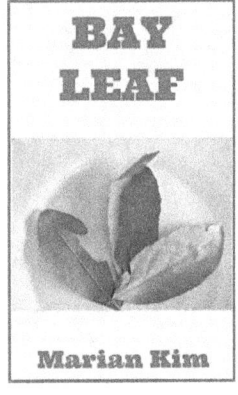

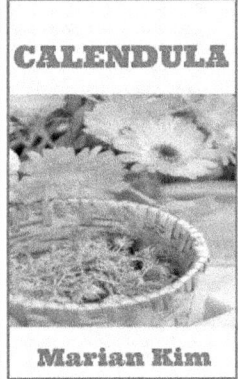

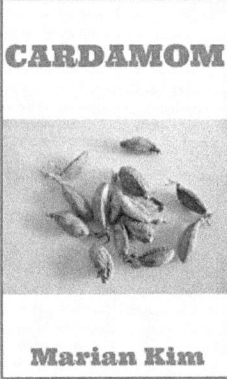

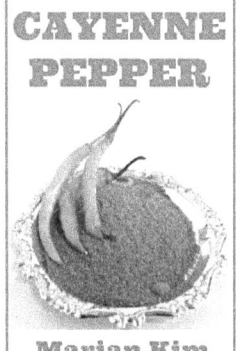

CAYENNE PEPPER

Marian Kim

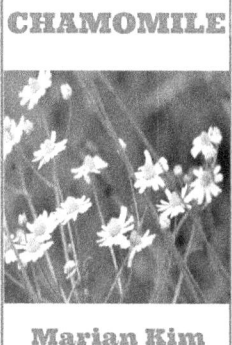

CHAMOMILE

Marian Kim

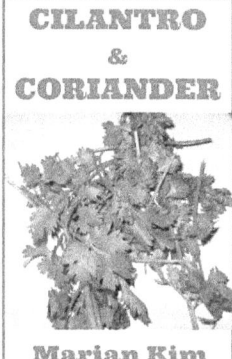

CILANTRO & CORIANDER

Marian Kim

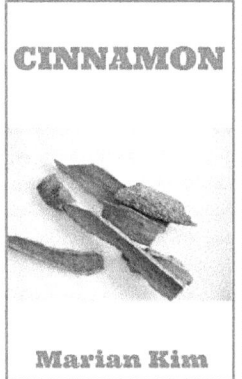

CINNAMON

Marian Kim

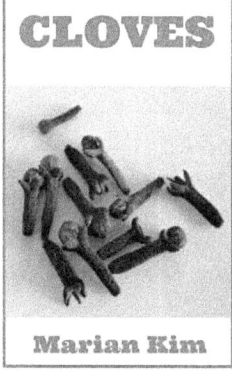

CLOVES

Marian Kim

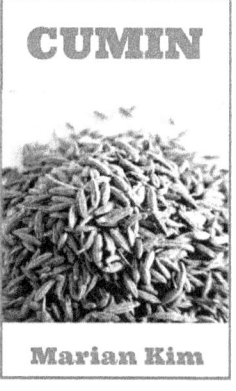

CUMIN

Marian Kim

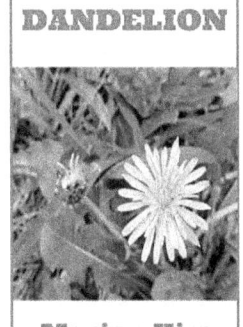

DANDELION

Marian Kim

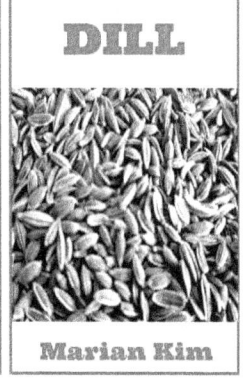

DILL

Marian Kim

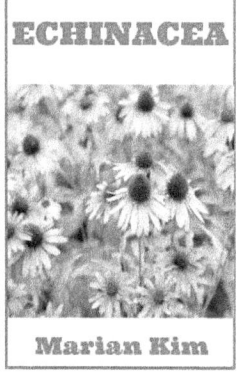

ECHINACEA

Marian Kim

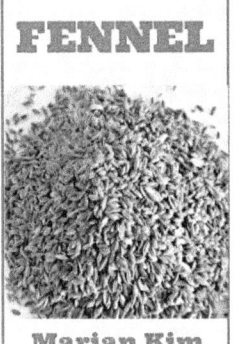

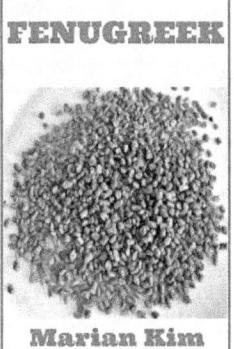

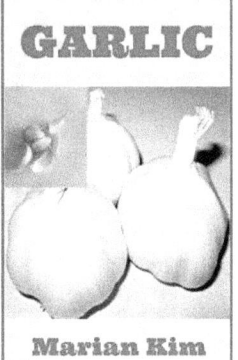

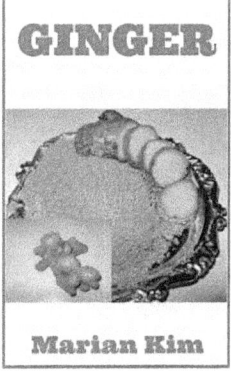

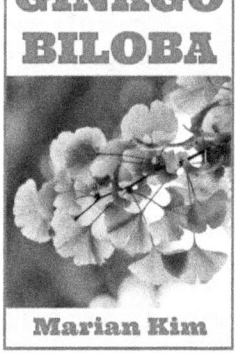

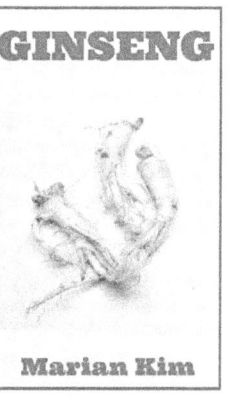

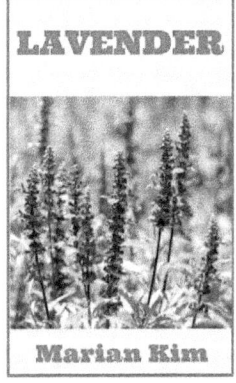

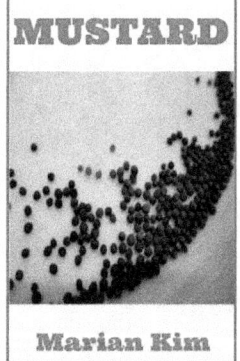

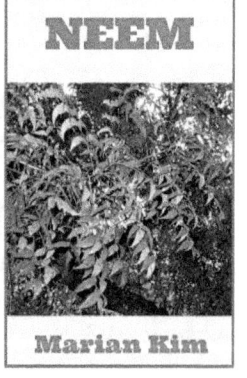

NUTMEG & MACE
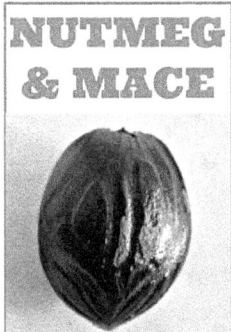
Marian Kim

OREGANO
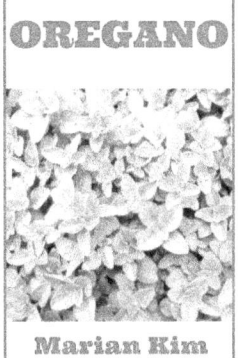
Marian Kim

PAPRIKA
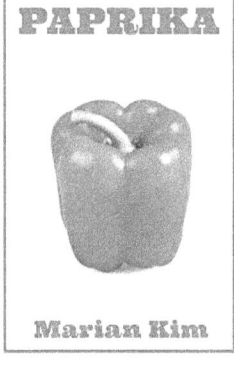
Marian Kim

PARSLEY
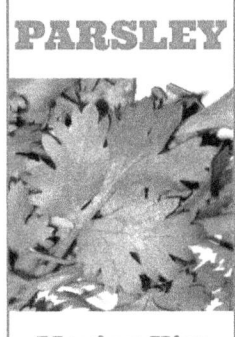
Marian Kim

BLACK & WHITE PEPPER
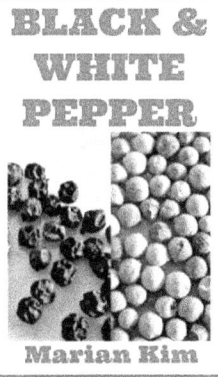
Marian Kim

PEPPERMINT
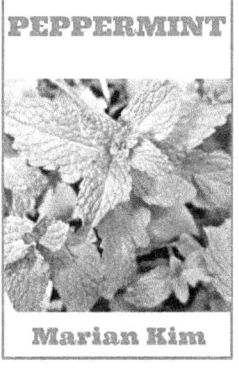
Marian Kim

ROSE HIPS
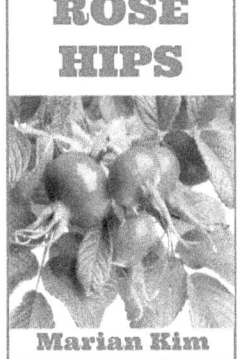
Marian Kim

ROSE PETALS
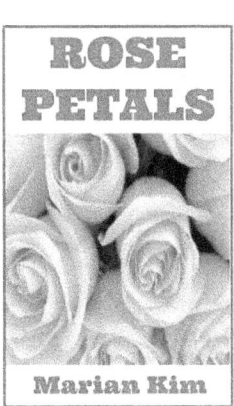
Marian Kim

ROSEMARY
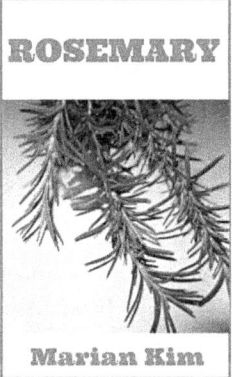
Marian Kim

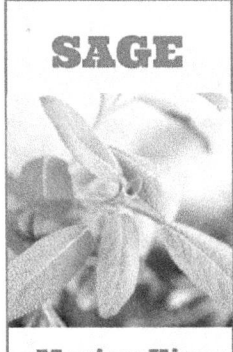

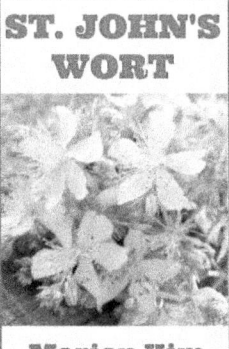

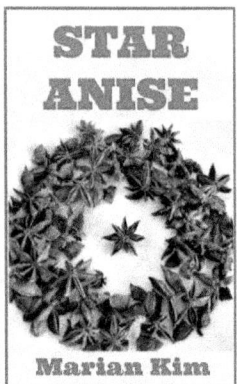

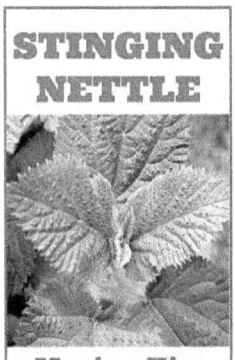

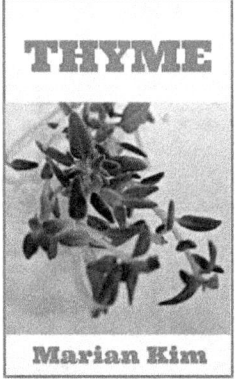

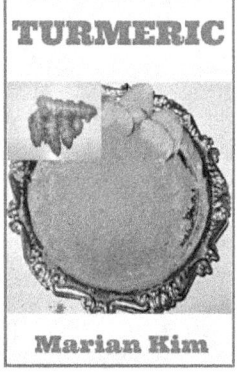

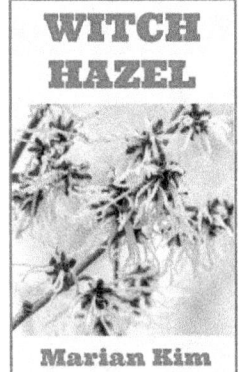

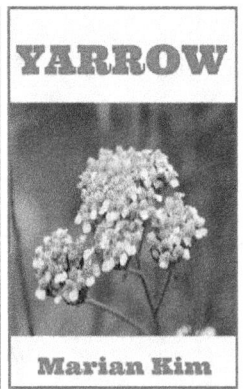

*****